MW01146384

Raw Food Diet: Delicious Raw Food Diet Tips
& Recipes to Revolutionize Your Health and (if desired) Start Losing Weight

By Marta Tuchowska

Copyright © 2014,2016 Marta Tuchowska

LEARN HOW TO INCORPORATE MORE RAW FOODS INTO YOUR DIET TO ENJOY HIGH ENERGY LEVELS, HOLISTIC WELLNESS, AND NATURAL WEIGHT LOSS.

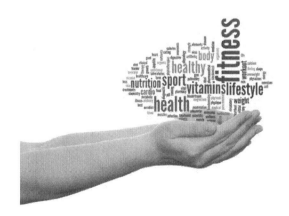

All information in this book has been carefully researched and checked for factual accuracy. However, the author and publishers make no warranty, expressed or implied, that the information contained herein is appropriate for every individual, situation or purpose, and assume no responsibility for errors or omission. The reader assumes the risk and full responsibility for all actions, and the author will not be held liable for any loss or damage, whether consequential, incidental, and special or otherwise, that may result from the information presented in this publication.

All cooking is an experiment in a sense, and many people come to the same or similar recipe over time. All recipes in this book have been derived from author's personal experience. Should any bear a close resemblance to those used elsewhere, that is purely coincidental.

The book is not intended to provide medical advice or to take the place of medical advice and treatment from your personal physician. Readers are advised to consult their own doctors or other qualified health professionals regarding the treatment of medical conditions. The author shall not be held liable or responsible for any misunderstanding or misuse of the information contained in this book. The information is not intended to diagnose, treat or cure any disease.

Contents

About This Book

Raw foods are a natural and delicious tool that can help you shed unwanted pounds, detoxify your body, concentrate better, and increase your energy levels.

This book is for you if...:

- you are interested in wellness, health, and naturopathy
- you want to increase your energy levels
- you wish to lose weight and detoxify
- you are a Paleo Diet fan and want to spice it up with raw foods and maybe add some variety into your diet (the recipes from this book are paleo-friendly)
- you are a vegan or vegetarian—this is an amazing raw foods party for you to be at!
- you are interested in super healthy and quick prep recipes
- you want to learn recipes that are flexible and can be adjusted to your current lifestyle and a diet
- you love healthy cooking in general and are interested in experimenting with new hot (even though they are raw and uncooked!) recipes

You don't have to go 100% vegan or vegetarian to enjoy the raw food diet benefits. I am really open-minded when it comes to different diets, their philosophies, and dietary lifestyles. I am not telling you what to do. I am not a guru. I am telling you what I do, so that I can hopefully inspire you to create your very own healthy and balanced nutritional lifestyle, so that you can feel great in your body. I am giving you information and inspiration, so that you can discover wellness through a balanced and holistic nutrition. Raw foods is one of the nutritional tools that I highly recommend.

I am sharing more than 50 amazingly delicious vegan-friendly raw foods recipes plus I am also giving plenty of cooking ideas for those of you guys who are not 100% vegan or vegetarian, so that you can combine my recipes with other diets or nutritional lifestyles that you may have chosen for yourself (for example, the Paleo Diet). My recipes are flexible and encourage creativity in cooking. It's up to you if you decide to do the raw food diet full-time or part-time. No matter which diet have you chosen for yourself and your family, it can be combined with more raw foods for more health and vitality.

It's all about adding...adding what? Fresh fruits and veggies!

Introduction

What is the biggest wellness and health obstacle that people are facing these days (apart from lack of time of course...)?

Lack of energy, yes! And if you lack energy, most likely you will miss on your other goals, like for example, working on your body or getting involved in other activities and projects that require energy and creativity.

Lack of energy means lack of enthusiasm and very often a sluggish mind and low concentration span. I have been there myself. From my own experience, I can tell you that if you feel that way, you usually tend to overindulge in unhealthy eating habits to make yourself feel better, at least for a while.

Health, on the other hand, attracts more health. If you get committed to wellness, and you start experiencing what transforming your body and mind feels like, you only want to carry on as it becomes your lifestyle.

I know that many people get a bit turned off when they hear the phrases like: "raw foods", "raw foodism", "going raw" as they immediately associate it with some massive sacrifice, going hungry, or eating "a rabbit's diet". Whereas it just does not work that way—incorporating raw foods into your diet is more energy, fun, natural weight loss aid, healthier body, and beautiful skin. These are the benefits that you can reap off by making at least 50% of your diet raw, clean foods.

Raw foods is one of the nutritional tools that I recommend, and I would define it as a highly therapeutic branch of naturopathy. I just look at it as natural medicine, something that can take care of your body and mind and nourish it properly.

Is It Another Fad Diet?

The raw foods as well as super foods are definitely very popular today, but I wouldn't call them a fad diet. In fact, this term was first coined in Switzerland at the end of the 19th century by a guy named Maximilian Bercher-Benner. He wasn't just "some guy"- he was a physician and a revolutionary holistic nutritionist. He was investigating the healing power of foods, something that at that time was rejected as an absurd. No one believed that nutrition could be like a medicine, other doctors laughed at Bercher-Benner, claiming that foods only serve to satisfy hunger, not to heal. If they had only known how mistaken they were!

Benner kept investigating and treating his patients with natural diets based on raw foods. He is actually the creator of muesli. If you are in Europe, you may have come across a muesli breakfast brand called after his name: "Bircher Muesli". I am not sure if this brand is also known on other continents.

Apart from the raw foods diet invention and investigation, Benner was also a believer in a regular physical activity and a balanced lifestyle. He believed that a body would heal itself if provided with all these healthy factors. He founded his own clinic, based in Zurich and he would help his patients gain more energy and zest for life as well as to lose weight, detoxify and fight allergies and other diseases.

Many other doctors would just laugh at his methods, but today, the model of his clinic inspires many wellness clinics and resorts. People pay big bucks for wellness retreats with yoga, raw foods, meditation, and a technology detox. Benner was definitely a wellness guru, and his teachings still serve us today.

The basic rundown of this simple diet is:

- The raw food diet, as the name suggests, promotes eating foods that are unprocessed and uncooked, such as fruits, vegetables, nuts, seeds, herbs.
- Some raw foodists, who are not vegan or vegetarian, also include some raw fish, eggs, as well as raw milk and fermented foods (unpasteurized) like for example, kefir or kombucha. Personally, when it comes to eating raw, I like the vegan approach as much as possible (and my recipes are focused on vegan raw foods).
- Raw foods are not necessarily 100% raw, some raw foodists cook their foods, but the basic rule is that the temperatures should not be higher than 40 degrees Celsius (or: 104 degrees Farenheit). Most of my recipes are 100% raw, but in some cases, I go through the slight cooking process.

6 simple reasons why raw foods are good for you:

- Excessive cooking kills the nutrients as well as many enzymes (these are responsible for proper digestion), and so if there are no raw foods in your diet, you are more likely to experience low energy levels and fatigue as well as sluggish digestion (after a cooked meal you usually feel sleepy, right?).
- Raw fruits and vegetables are an excellent sources of natural dietary fiber, hence the natural weight loss benefit.
- Raw foods will nourish your body with tons of vitamins and minerals that are crucial for beautiful skin and hair
- You will strenghten your immune system

More benefits of raw foods:

- easy to prepare
- excellent source of energy for the summer
- can be combined with any other diet that you have chosen to follow
- provide you with endless possibilities as for tasty and sweet desserts, and can help you control food cravings.

Let me give you my personal opinion before we get to the facts, and of course, the recipes. This is a practical recipe book for modern people who would like to experiment a little bit with "raw-fooding" and increase their energy levels and quality of life. I am not telling you to go vegan or raw-food 100% (unless you want to, then I will give you all my support), just like I am not telling you to follow a given diet. I am trying to encourage you to create your own healthy nutrition habits. The raw foods is one of the tools that I would like to explain in this book. Your homework will be to find your own way and see what works for you.

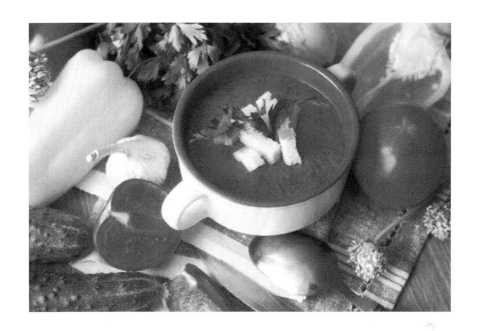

Disclaimer

A physician has not written the information contained in this book. Before making any drastic changes to your diet, consult your physician first. Adding more raw foods to your diet can be a great natural tool for health, energy and wellness, but the author is not making any claims, this book should never be a substitute for any professional or medical treatments.

Frequently Asked Questons

My personal opinion on raw foods will be reflected in the following questions that I very often get asked:

- *Does going on a raw foods diet mean that I will only be able eat raw foods all the time?*

This is totally up to you. Try adding more and more raw foods into your diet or at least reduce the cooking process, and eliminate the "overcooking" process (more than 30-40 degrees Celsius) as much as possible. Some people do raw foods full-time, some of them do it part-time. I believe that it also depends on your geographical location or a season.

- *Is the Raw Foods Diet the same as the Alkaline Diet?*

No, even though these 2 diets very often overlap, and many Alkaline people are into raw foods, just like many raw foodists are into Alkalinity, these are 2 different diets.

Not all raw foods are super alkaline just like not all the alkaline foods are raw. I do the alkaline diet, and I have some cooked meals in my diet as well, but I don't overdo this process. It is also worth mentioning that consuming too many cooked foods is acid forming. Hence, there are many alkaline people, like me, who try to eat more and more raw foods to achieve their alkaline wellness dream.

Those who follow the alkaline diet, are mostly interested in choosing raw fruits and vegetables that have strong alkalizing effect, such as: all green vegetables, tomatoes, lemons, garlic, onions, grapefruits (more alkaline tips in my recipes!)

- *At this stage of my life, I can't really make a decision to go vegan or vegetarian. Am I still able to do the raw foods?*

Yes, everyone can add more raw foods into their diet, it's as simple as that. I know many people who follow the Paleo Diet, and they realized they were consuming too much meat (the typical eggs with bacon thing!). By adding more fresh raw foods into their diet, they were able to achieve a healthy balance.

And if you decide to go vegan or vegetarian—congratulations! I think that this decision comes from one's heart. I know that in order to do it the right way, one must learn at least the basics of nutrition and make sure that the vegan/vegetarian lifestyle they follow gives their body all the nutrients.

- *Is the Raw Foods Diet the same as the Paleo Diet?*

No, the raw foods (except from kefir and raw milk of course) are Paleo-friendly. This means that if you are Paleo, all the raw fruits and vegetables (even raw fish if you decide to choose this path) is acceptable with your Paleolithic lifestyle.

Many scientists claim that back in the Paleolithic era, our ancestors would mostly eat raw foods, which makes sense (maybe they were so exhausted and hungry after hunting and gathering that they did not have enough energy to gather around the fire? Who knows?), however, the Raw Foods and

Paleo are too different things. Most of the raw-foodists are strictly vegan, and so I am not too sure if they would develop friendly feelings towards carnivorous Paleos...

- *I am a bit skeptical about the raw food diets as I am not that spiritual, and I heard that the raw food followers involve too much spirituality in all this stuff. I just want to lose weight and detoxify. Can I still do it?*

First of all, everyone is on a different journey. People may have different beliefs, passions and dreams and we should respect all of them. You just need to focus on yourself- stop comparing yourself to others. Do what's right for you...Listen to your body.

Just concentrate on your health goals, and apply the raw foods as much as you can. Detoxification and weight loss will come naturally. And, if doing this raw foods process, you observe any other changes, maybe in your behavior, outlook on life, emotions, and spirituality that positively impact your life— spread the real word of health and wellness. Be curious about what you do. See it as a journey. There is nothing wrong with starting a raw food diet simply because you want to lose weight. It's your journey and your motivation. Use it as a fuel that propels you mentally and emotionally.

OK, back to the questions!

- *I am a vegetarian, but not a vegan. I consume cheese and dairy occasionally. The same with eggs—I like free range eggs, and I have about 2-3 of them a week. Is my lacto-vegetarian lifestyle compatible with the raw foods diet?*

Yes, like I mentioned earlier, everyone can add more raw foods into their diet, and you don't have to a full-time vegan raw-food diet if it is not for you. Just combine it with your current diet. You may also be interested to learn that not all raw-foodists are vegan. There are different schools of a raw foods diet, and some of them allow consuming raw, unpasteurized milk or kefir, the same with eggs and some kinds of cheese. This is why you can combine raw foods easily with your current vegetarian lifestyle.

- *How can I lose weight using raw foods? What does eating raw have to do with weight loss?*

Weight loss is like a secondary effect of eating a raw foods diet (at least 70% raw foods). You will give your body more fiber and will also have more energy levels and, so you will be able to work more on your body. You will experience this natural motivation boost thanks to increased energy levels. You will also be able to detoxify your body and heal it from the inside out.

- *You say that raw foods are vegetarian and vegan and are good for weight loss. I am skeptical. I went vegetarian and even vegan for a few years and instead of losing weight, I gained on weight. Isn't it just another fad?*

I totally understand how you feel. I also had the same problem in the past, but the mistake that I made is that I did not learn enough about vegan and vegetarian friendly nutrition. I used to abuse pasta, rice, and bread and did not have much variety in my diet. I eliminated meat but did not anything about how to combine other foods to obtain natural protein. I had no idea what foods like "quinoa" were. I also did not consume enough raw fruits and vegetables.

I am sure that you can do it right this time, and if you add more raw foods into your diet, weight loss will be like a secondary effect alongside other health benefits I have already mentioned. Of course, when it comes to weight loss, it's not only about diet. You must work out regularity. This is what works for me—I know that if I don't go to the gym regularity, I will put on weight.

Raw foods will help you revitalize and recover after excessive workouts. There is a myriad of options when it comes to healthy before and after workouts vegan, raw food smoothies.

Finally—are the raw foods safe?

Yes, of course they are, they are like a natural medicine.

However, (and a very big "HOWEVER"), if you are new to a vegan or semi-vegan lifestyle, and your current diet is far from healthy, or you suffer from any serious health problem or condition, are on medication, pregnant, or lactating-consulting your doctor first is a must. If this is a new thing for you, and it is much different to what your body is used to, I absolutely recommend you get regular blood tests just to see if you are getting enough nutrients and vitamins. And again, see your doctor or a natural health professional before trying any new nutritional patterns.

In my opinion, everyone can do the raw foods diet, but what works for me may not work for you. People are very often too concerned about jumping on a given bandwagon, instead of creating a nutritional lifestyle that will suit their needs based on different factors like: age, sex, occupation, climatic zone, possible illnesses, activity, and eating preferences. What also does matter is where you are now with your nutritional habits.

For example, if you know that you eat junk food, or processed foods all the time, you might consider doing a cleanse program, but if you are already healthy, or more-or-less healthy and balanced, I would not worry about going overboard. Just add more raw foods, or even better, alkaline raw foods on a regular basis, so that you can experience more energy levels, lose some weight, and just feel better in your body.

The Raw Foods & the Alkaline Diet

Like I already explained, not all raw foods are alkaline. People very often think that all fruits and vegetables are alkaline, but if you have a look at the following "mini charts", you will see that some fruits are slightly acid-forming (because of their high sugar content)

ALKALINE VEGETABLES AND FRUIT:

- Asparagus
- Basil
- Cauliflower
- Carrots
- Beetroots
- Eggplants
- Garlic
- Onions
- Parsley
- Celery
- Cucumber
- Broccoli
- Pepper
- Zucchini
- Spinach
- Kale
- Wakame
- Pumpkin
- Radish
- Squashes
- Endive
- Cabbage
- Ginger
- Alfalfa
- Watercress
- Lettuce
- Avocado
- Tomato
- Lemon
- Lime

- Grapefruit
- Fresh Coconut
- Pomegranate

ACID-FORMING FFUITS (IF YOU WANT TO KEEP IT ALKALINE, REDUCE TO 30% OF YOUR DIET, but first of all, see what works for you):

- Grapes
- Tropical Fruits
- Cantaloupe
- Cranberries
- Currants
- Mango
- Apple
- Apricot
- Currants
- Dates
- Bananas
- Peach
- Pear
- Honeydew Melon
- Orange
- Pineapple
- Plum
- Prunes
- Raisins
- Raspberries
- Strawberries

Most veggies are alkaline (from mildly alkaline as, for example, broccoli and kale, to mildly alkaline as, for example, pumpkin). Olives are acid-forming, all fermented foods are (still, I love them in salads!). When I grab some raw foods, I tend to care about the nutrients and vitamins that they provide my body with, but I also want to maintain a healthy alkaline balance as this is what works for me and for my wellbeing (70% alkaline-forming foods is enough).

Of course, processed junk food is extremely acid-forming and should be eliminated completely from your diet. No matter which healthy diet have you chosen for yourself, processed junk food must go... I don't even want to hear about any excuses here.

Raw foods can help you eliminate all that processed junk; you will see that my raw recipes are exciting, delicious, and fun. They will satisfy your taste buds and nourish your body and mind. A body that does not lack any nutrients won't ask you to indulge in unhealthy foods. A body that lacks nutrients will send you "I am hungry" signals, and this is one of the reasons (aside from emotional factors of course) that people go binging.

When do I go on raw foods?

I really enjoy raw foods during the summer, especially during the day when it's really hot. They give me energy, vitamins, and minerals that I tend to sweat out (it's really hot here in the summer). So that's the climate factor.

I don't do raw foods full-time. I do them part-time (about 70%, sometimes less, sometimes more than that) as this is what works for me. This means that I also combine the raw foods diet with other diets that I find healthy (for example, the Mediterranean diet and the Macrobiotic diet). I also eat cooked (but not overcooked) and steamed foods, but I know when to get back to raw foods. Over the years, I developed the skill of listening to my body and observing how it reacts to given foods. I take into consideration my digestive system, my nervous system, my energy levels, and my concentration.

How to create your own healthy nutrition bandwagon and be the driver?

It's easy—just get enough knowledge and inspiration and see what works for you. In case of raw foods, start adding more raw foods recipes to your diet and observe what's happening. For me, this is an excellent holistic wellness tool that I get hooked on in the summer. I also eat raw foods in the winter, but quite naturally, my body craves something like cooked foods and soups. I give my body what it needs.

So let's get started. As you can see, my dear reader, I try to be open-minded about different diets (as long as these are no fads!), and I think of them as different wellness tools to create a healthy body you deserve.

Yet, when it comes to diets, many people think that it has to be all or nothing...I want to give you freedom from this limiting belief (yes, it is a limiting belief).

Baby steps always work! Focus on adding...adding more raw foods into your diet. Enjoy the process of making fresh, colorful smoothies and salads. See it as a game!

One more thing—to be honest, I hate the word "diet". Let's call is a "lifestyle" OK? Yea, that sounds better!

****

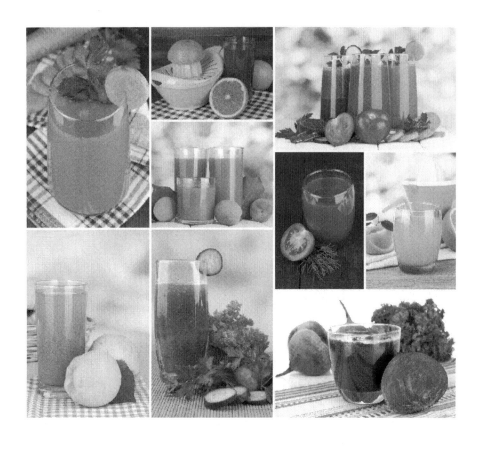

Recipe Measurements

I love keeping ingredient measurements as simple as possible-this is why I stick to tablespoons, teaspoons and cups.

The cup measurement I use is the American cup measurement. I also use it for dry ingredients. If you are new to it, let me help you:

If you don't have American Cup measures, just use a metric or imperial liquid measuring jug and fill your jug with your ingredient to the corresponding level. Here's how to go about it:

1 American Cup= 250ml= 8 fl.oz

For example:

If a recipe calls for 1 cup of almonds, simply place your almonds into your measuring jug until it reaches the 250 ml/8oz mark.

I know that different countries use different measurements and I wanted to make things simple for you.

Translations (US-UK English)

Eggplant=Aubergine

Zucchini=Courgette

Cilantro=Coriander

Garbanzo Beans=Chickpeas

Navy Beans-=Haricot Beans

Aragula=Rocket

Broth=Stock

Raw Food Recipes

RECIPE #1 Alkaline-Southern European

Tomatoes and cucumbers are extremely alkaline. Whether you follow the alkaline diet or not, you can reap their benefits, alkalinize your system, and give your body many vital minerals and vitamins. This recipe is really easy and quick to prepare.

Perfect for quick lunch in the summer, or as a snack. It is suitable for vegans, vegetarians, Paleo enthusiasts, alkaline diet lovers, and also those who follow the low-cholesterol, traditional Mediterranean diet!

Check it out for yourself!

Serves-2

Ingredients

- 3 cucumbers
- 5 ripe tomatoes
- 2 tablespoons of basil oil (you can make it yourself; just mix some chopped basil with some olive oil, and leave overnight in a dark bottle. You're going to obtain some really delicious basil oil!)
- 1 tablespoon chopped basil
- ¼ cup black olives
- Himalaya salt
- pepper
- 1 garlic clove

Preparation

*If you wish to prepare some basil oil, just for this occasion, in a bowl, place two tablespoons of olive oil along with the chopped basil and let marinate one hour. Personally, for practical reasons, I prefer to do things in bulk, this is why I use the way I presented in the ingredients section—I do the whole bottle of basil oil to have it ready when I am on the go...

1. Wash and peel the tomatoes, remove the seeds, and chop into small squares.

2. Peel cucumbers and cut into thin slices.

3. Remove the pits from the olives.

4. Peel the garlic clove and chop finely.

5. Mix all the ingredients in a bowl, add some basil oil, and add pepper and salt to taste. Garnish with some chopped basil.

Enjoy!

RECIPE#2 Refreshing Spinach Smoothie

This is a really easy to prepare green smoothie that will give you both some nice refreshment and energy. I like to have it with my salads as a refreshing drink or even as a dessert.

Serves -2

Ingredients

- 2 cups of spinach
- 4 peeled apples
- A small handful of fresh mint
- 1 cup of water

Preparation

- Wash the spinach and mint.
- Peel the apples.
- Place all ingredients in a blender and add some water. Blend
- Serve immediately. I like to add a few ice cubes and some cinnamon.

RECIPE#3 Herbal Dip

This recipe is another example of alkaline raw foods. I love to have this refreshing dips with some cucumber or carrot sticks. Eating healthy is just so awesome.

Serves-2

Ingredients

- 4 tomatoes
- 2 onions
- 2 big red peppers
- 4 garlic cloves
- 2 tablespoons soaked chia seeds
- 2 tablespoons of olive oil
- Himalaya salt
- Thyme, basil, sage, oregano (I use 1 teaspoon of each)
- ½ cup walnuts or other nuts

Preparation

1. Soak the walnuts and tomatoes for about 8 hours.
2. Peel the onion and garlic, and mince them.
3. Cut the pepper into small pieces.
4. Chop the thyme, basil, and other herbs.
5. Drain and grind the walnuts to a paste.
6. Drain the tomatoes and cut into very small chunks.
7. In a bowl, place the chopped walnuts, onion, garlic, bell pepper, tomatoes, herbs, oil, chia, and salt, and mix to a paste (you can use a food processor to make it nice and smooth).
8. Optional: cool down in a fridge for about an hour.

9. Serve with some raw veggies as a dip. So yummy and spicy!

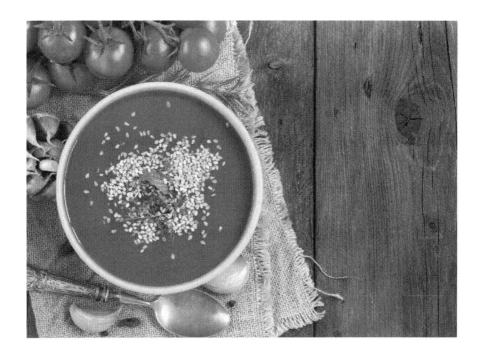

RECIPE #4 Watercress Raw Pesto

It's very important to make the raw food diet as tasty as possible. This will make you naturally hooked on it, and so you will crave more raw foods. This is another example of a pesto-dip style like dish. If you want to make it 100% raw, have it with some raw veggies or as a salad dressing.

Serves:2-3

Ingredients

- 2 cloves of garlic
- sea salt
- 1 tablespoon pine nuts (soaked in water for a few hours)
- 4 walnuts (soaked in water for a few hours)
- 6 leaves of basil
- 8 tomatoes, peeled
- ½ cup of fresh watercress (washed and dried)
- 2 tablespoons of olive oil

Preparation

1. Crush the garlic cloves with two pinches of sea salt, pine nuts, and walnuts.

2. Place the mix into a bowl. Add the chopped basil and olive oil.

3. Finally, add tomatoes, mix well, and blend in a blender or food processor.

4. Stir well and serve. Enjoy!

More suggestions:

You can also have it with some steamed zucchinis, or if you do the raw food diet part-time, you can have it with some gluten-free pasta, brown rice, quinoa, or cus-cus. The list goes on and on!

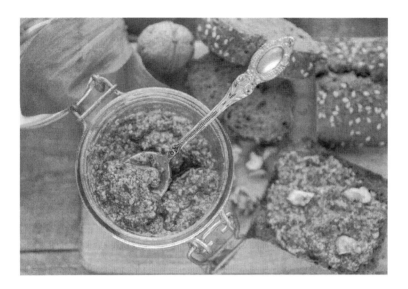

RECIPE#5 Raw Alkaline Salad with a Sweet Twist!

I eat at least one salad a day. In the summertime, I love to have salads for lunch. Creativity is the key. For example, I knew that beetroots were good for me, but had no idea how to make them tasty. This salad is the result of my experiments. I love how different blend. For example tastes, you have onions and radishes that are a bit hot, and then you have some raisins and beetroot that make it sweet.

Serves: 2-3
Ingredients

- ¼ cup of extra virgin olive oil
- 1 piece of ginger root about 1 cm
- 1 lemon
- 2 small endives
- 1 cup of watercress
- 1 cup of oak leaf lettuce
- 1 large raw beetroot
- 2 carrots
- Half red onion
- 1 cup of radishes
- ¼ cup of raisins
- sea salt or Himalaya salt

Preparation

1. Peel the ginger, slice, and dice. Put it in a small pan with half a lemon skin (reserve pulp to squeeze), and cover with oil. Bring to low heat (lower than 40 Celsius)

for 15 minutes, remove from heat, cover, and let it cool down. This is going to be our super tasty dressing!

2. In the meantime, wash the leaves of endive, watercress, and lettuce and dry.

3. Peel the beets and cut into very thin sheets.

4. Peel the carrots and cut into thin slices; also slice radishes.

5. Cut the onion into thin rings.

6. Mix all the ingredients in a bowl, add some olive oil, lemon juice, and a few pinches of salt.

7. Add the beets, sliced carrot, radish, onion, and raisins. Pour on the dressing (the one from the step 1.), mix, and serve immediately!

Enjoy!

RECIPES #6 Sweet Raw!

Here comes a really nice and sweet fruity recipe. Most of the ingredients, even though raw and healthy, are not really that alkaline (except for tomatoes, almonds, and lemons that help balance this recipe). The reason why I make this comment is just for you to learn that not all raw foods are alkaline (very often, people use the terms "raw" and "alkaline" as if they meant the same thing, which is really confusing). However, if you are interested in following the alkaline diet, don't get discouraged, these ingredients can still form part of about 30% of your diet. This salad is delicious and nutritious. I love to have it when I crave sweets!

Serves: 3-4

Ingredients

- 1 large mango
- 4 figs
- 10 cherry tomatoes
- 1 cup of grapes
- 4 kiwis
- 2 Pears
- 4 tablespoons of fresh currants
- 1 cup of fresh blueberries
- ¼ cup of almonds
- Juice of 1 lemon

Preparation

1. Wash the fruits and peel.
2. Cut all the fruits in small pieces.

3. Blend the blueberries with some lemon juice.
4. Mix all the ingredients, and add the blueberry cream.
5. Garnish with some almonds.

Enjoy!

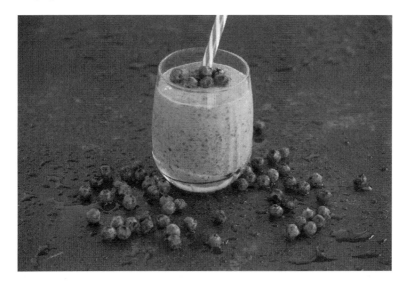

RECIPE #7 Your Raw Vitamins

This is an excellent raw shake full of vitamins and minerals. I love it before and after my workouts!

Serves: 2

Ingredients

- ¼ of white cabbage
- 4 apples
- 2 avocadoes
- 1 cup of coconut water
- Some ginger to spice it up

Preparation

1. Wash the ingredients.
2. Peel the apple.
3. Peel and pit avocado.
4. Cut the cabbage into small pieces.
5. Blend until smooth.
6. Garnish with a slice of lemon or lime.

So delicious and revitalizing!

RECIPE #8 Agar-agar Salad

Here comes another creative salad recipe. I love algae, and I think that once you start using them and realize that it's so easy to prepare, and at the same time, really good for you, you will get addicted to them.

Carrots are excellent summer foods, they will help you make your skin look healthier (beta-carotene), and they are perfect for pale complexions!

Apples and carrots are, in my opinion, an excellent combination!

Serves: 3-4

Ingredients

- 6 carrots
- ½ cup of of hazelnuts
- Half of red cabbage
- 2 tablespoons of agar-agar algae
- 1 cup of green mustard sprouts
- 6 tomatoes
- 3 garlic cloves
- 2 apples
- Juice of 2 lemons
- 3 tablespoons of olive oil

Preparation

1. Peel carrots and cut into strips, sprinkle with some lemon juice.

2. Soak agar-agar seaweed in some filtered water (for about 10 mins).

3. In the meantime, cut the cabbage into thin strips.

4. Chop the hazelnuts.

5. Drain the agar-agar seaweed.

For the dressing

1. Soak the tomatoes, and remove the peel

2. Peel the garlic and apples

3. Place all ingredients in a blender, and blend until a smooth cream.

4. Mix all the ingredients in a bowl, and add the dressing. Sprinkle over some olive oil mixed with lemon juice. Serve immediately.

RECIPE #9 Orange Salad

I used to think that mixing oranges with onions or garlic was nothing more than a sign of going mad. A few years ago, when I was in Italy, an Italian friend of mine, introduced me to a similar recipe that he said was a traditional Sicilian salad. I have transformed it a bit and added a few ingredients. If you are looking for a quick, detoxifying salad, just mix some oranges with a little bit of garlic, onions, lemon juice, and herbs like basil. If you would like to make it more complex, just follow this recipe of mine:

Serves: 2

Ingredients:

- 4 oranges
- 4 square inches of wakame seaweed
- 1 ½ large fennel.
- Lemon juice
- Olive oil
- 2 avocados
- 1 clove of Garlic and ginger (more or less the same amount)
- ½ onion

Preparation:

For the dressing

- Peel and pit avocados
- Peel the garlic and ginger
- Place the avocados, garlic and ginger in a blender, add some water and olive oil and blend. Add some Himalaya salt and black pepper to taste.

For the salad:

1. Soak wakame seaweed in filtered water, for about 15 mins.
2. Peel the oranges and cut into slices
3. Cut the petals of fennel and get the heart.
4. Cut the fennel into small pieces.
5. Place the fennel in a bowl and sprinkle with sea salt and add some   lemon juice and add algae.
6. Add the oranges, and mix them with onion(finely chopped).
7. Serve with the avocado dressing. Sprinkle over some lemon juice to spice it up. Enjoy!

RECIPE#10 Green Alkaline Raw Salad

This is a great, quick salad recipe, and it's recommended for those who are concerned about their pH balancing. Let's make it raw and alkaline!

Serves: 3

Ingredients

- 2 cucumbers
- 1 cup of spinach
- 1 onion
- 1 garlic clove
- 1 cup of radishes
- Half of iceberg lettuce
- ¼ cup of raw almonds
- Black pepper
- 1 tablespoon of fresh basil or rosemary
- ¼cup of coconut milk or sweet almond milk
- 2 tablespoons of olive oil
- Juice of 1 lemon

Preparation

For the dressing

- Mix about ¼ cup of coconut milk or sweet almond milk with some olive oil (about 2 tablespoons), juice of 1 lemon, fresh herbs (basil or rosemary), and 1 garlic clove (finely chopped). Add some pepper and Himalaya salt to taste.

For the salad

1. Wash the cucumbers, spinach, radishes, onion, and lettuce.
2. Peel the cucumbers and cut into small pieces.
3. Cut the spinach and iceberg lettuce.
4. Cut the radishes and onion, and mix with other ingredients.
5. Add the raw almonds and the dressing.
6. Serve immediately, enjoy!

RECIPE#11 Apple and Carrot Easy Salad

This is a classic apple and carrot salad that is very popular where I am originally from. I have transformed this simple recipe with a few extra ingredients.

OPTION 1. If you feel like something sweet...

Serves 2-3
Ingredients:
- 4 apples
- 4 carrots
- ¼ cup of raisins
- A few dates
- 1 teaspoon of cinnamon
- 1 tablespoon of coconut milk

Instructions:
1. Wash and peel the apples and carrots.
2. Grate the apples and carrots.
3. In a bowl, mix with some raisins and dates. Add coconut milk and cinnamon.
4. Optional: sprinkle over some lemon juice and add a few almonds.
5. Enjoy! It's so healthy and delicious!

OPTION 2. If you want to make it spicy...

Serves-2
Ingredients:
- 4 apples
- 4 carrots

- 1 garlic clove
- Half onion
- Pinch of Himalaya salt
- Pinch of curry
- Pinch of pepper or chili
- Juice of half lemon
- Olive oil

Instructions

1. Wash and peel the apples and carrots.
2. Grate the apples and carrots.
3. Cut the garlic and onion into tiny pieces—you can also grate them.
4. Mix all the ingredients in a bowl, add salt, curry, and pepper (or chili) to taste. Sprinkle over some lemon juice and olive oil.

Serve immediately! Enjoy!

OPTIONAL: if you want to transform this recipe and add something that is not raw foodie, then I suggest you add some cooked lentils (cool them down after cooking). So delicious!

OPTION3. Anti-oxidant and Alkaline
Serves-2
Ingredients:
- 4 apples
- 4 carrots
- 1 garlic clove
- 2 cucumbers
- 2 tomatoes
- Pinch of Himalaya salt
- Juice of half lemon

- Olive oil

Instructions:
1. Wash and peel the apples and carrots.
2. Grate them.
3. Wash and peel the cucumber and tomatoes, slice them.
4. Mix all the ingredients in a bowl. Add some minced garlic, olive oil, and freshly squeezed lemon juice and Himalaya salt. So delicious and healthy!

RECIPE#12 Raw Breakfast Muesli

This is just a classic of raw foods breakfasts!

It's very easy and quick to prepare and will help you start a day with optimal energy levels!

Serves 2-3

Ingredients

- 4 cups of raw almond milk
- 1 banana
- 1 avocado
- 1 cup of nuts and seeds mix (I mix almonds with sunflower seeds)
- Juice of 1 lemon

OPTIONAL: 3-4 ripe grapefruits to squeeze the juice to accompany the muesli breakfast (grapefruits are really alkaline and are excellent source of vitamin C!)

Instructions

1. Wash and peel the banana and avocado, and slice them.
2. In a bowl, mix with raw almond milk and the mix of nuts.
3. Add some lemon juice.
4. Serve immediately with some grapefruit juice if you want to keep it alkaline!
5. OPTIONAL: sprinkle over some cinnamon and spiruline powder.

This recipe is not only for breakfast, it is also an excellent mid-afternoon snack!

RECIPE#13 Kale Wraps

There are plenty of ways that you can create your own, super healthy and raw kale wraps. These are rich in natural chlorophyll that form part of a balanced, alkaline diet.

Serves-2

Ingredients

- A few big kale leaves
- 1 onion
- 1 garlic clove
- 2 tomatoes
- 2 avocados
- 1 cucumber
- Crashed almonds
- Himalaya salt

Instructions

1. Wash and peel the veggies.
2. Blend the tomatoes with onion, garlic, and avocado. Add some crashed almonds (about 4 teaspoons).
3. Peel and slice the cucumber and mix with the blended ingredients.
4. Add some Himalaya salt to taste.
5. Spread the filling on each kale leaf and make wraps.

Sprinkle over some lemon juice and enjoy!

RECIPE#14 Anti-oxidant Salad

I know that the combination of ingredients may seem more than weird, but as soon as you try it, you will begin to love it. I have created this recipe one evening when I really fancied a salad, but at the same time, did not feel like going shopping for particular ingredients. Salads are so easy as long as you use your imagination!

Serves-2

Ingredients

- 2 grapefruits
- 2 carrots
- 2 cucumbers
- 1 garlic clove
- Half of onion
- 2 tomatoes
- 1 avocado
- Juice of 1 lemon

Instructions

1. Wash and peel the fruits and veggies.
2. Slice the carrots, tomatoes, cucumbers.
3. Pit the avocado and cut into small pieces.
4. Slice the grapefruits.
5. Mix all the ingredients in a bowl, and sprinkle over some fresh lemon juice!

RECIPE#15 Mediterranean Salad

Another great salad recipe inspired by the Mediterranean Diet!

Serves-2

Ingredients

- Half of iceberg salad
- 1 cup of cherry tomatoes
- 1 cup of green olives, pitted
- 1 cup of black olives, pitted
- 1 red pepper
- 1 onion
- 2 carrots
- Olive oil
- Juice of 1 lemon
- Balsamic vinegar

Instructions

1. Wash all the ingredients. Let the iceberg lettuce dry (leave it on a clean kitchen cloth or in a sieve).
2. Cut the cherry tomatoes in two.
3. Slice the onion, red pepper, and carrots.
4. Slice the iceberg lettuce.
5. Mix with other ingredients and add some olive oil (about 2 tablespoons), lemon juice, and balsamic vinegar.

OPTIONAL: if you are not a vegan or vegetarian, you can also add some tuna or raw shrimp to this salad. Remember that tuna is not a part of the raw foods diet (canned tuna is cooked). I just mention this option if you wish to do a part time raw foods diet or mix it with other options, diets, and tools. It's totally up to you!

RECIPE#16 Amazing Citrus Salad

I know that eating raw lemons seems like a bad idea, but if you manage to combine it with something sweeter, the whole process will be both healthy and pleasurable. This is a recipe inspired by the old naturopathic remedy to prevent colds and it includes eating lemons with honey (this is what my grandparents taught me!). However, honey is not a vegan product. It's raw, but it's not vegan. This is why I added a vegan option which is maple syrup or stevia.

Many people take artificial vitamin C, and I believe that in most cases such supplements are not necessary to take. These are synthetic vitamins that you should avoid, unless, your doctor tells you to take them because you have some deficiency in your system. Still, in my opinion, you can just add more natural vitamin C foods to your diet.

Yesterday I saw someone's video on YouTube, and the guy was telling people to buy vitamin C supplements (along plenty of other pills and powders for weight loss and muscle gain), the same he was apparently using every day (it's called affiliate marketing!); he was even saying that one can't go wrong with vitamin C as it is impossible to overdose because it's a vitamin. Ok, you can't overdose on natural vitamin C, but if you stick to artificial supplements, especially when your body does not really need it, you can do damage your liver and kidneys. Again, these supplements are big money for marketers. Holistic health practitioners like me, and also medical doctors may have different opinion.

So, to sum up, if you want to take any vitamin supplements, don't do it, until you have consulted with your doctor first. All marketers and big companies will tell you that you need to take those if you are active and pressed for time, but let me tell you one thing- I am active, and I hardly ever take breaks. I just love what I do and it keeps me alive. I do take care about my nutrition in a holistic way. I get blood tests and checkups regularly (I usually choose doctors who, aside from their formal medical education also do naturopathy, if you have read my other books, I am sure you remember me talking about naturopathic doctors) and to be honest, I don't need to take any artificial vitamins.

Nature is abundant in everything that you need. Don't self-medicate with artificial vitamins (unless, like I said earlier, you have a certain medical condition and your doctor, physician or any medical professional tells you to do so). Avoid internet gurus, also those from YouTube. They "recommend" certain products that they may not be even using themselves, only because if you buy them from their links, they get a commission from their affiliate marketing (I have nothing against ethical affiliate marketing by the way!). So, don't get brainwashed and be careful where you spend your hard earned money on. Then, of course, also be careful about your body and the possible harm that some synthetic supplements can do to you if abused.

Ok, back to the recipes!

Try this recipe on a regular basis, especially in the winter time. In my climate zone, I like to use it regularly after the end of summer, when temperatures start going lower.

We need vitamin C for proper iron absorption as well. This is why it is also recommended for those who are iron deficient.

If you are interested in natural supplements, I recommend good quality royal jelly. If you can get it raw, it will taste as sweet as honey, and you could also use it with this recipe! Again, remember that honey is not suitable for vegans.

Serves-2

Ingredients

- 4 lemons
- 1 garlic clove
- 1 cup of baby spinach
- 2 oranges
- A few tablespoons of maple syrup or stevia
- Or (if you are not vegan)-A few tablespoons of raw organic honey (you can also add some raw royal jelly, check the daily doses according to the manufacturer's instructions)
- ¼ cup of raisins

Instructions:

1. Wash and peel the lemons and oranges. Slice them and cut into small pieces.
2. Wash the spinach, cut, and mix with lemons and oranges.
3. Sprinkle over some raisins and maple syrup or honey.
4. Serve immediately! This is natural vitamin C! It can help you achieve wellness and be healthier without spending big bucks.

RECIPE#17 Raw Oats with a Twist

I often get asked if oats or porridge are on or off the raw foods diets. The answer is very simple, as long as the oats are not processed and were not cooked in any way, they are raw and perfectly fine. The way I prepare them in the summer is to make them nice and refreshing, this is why I spice them up with some fruits.

I like raw Scottish oats, I always make sure they are organic. I got hooked on them when living in the UK. Oats can be one of the quickest and the healthiest breakfasts ever.

Serves-2

Ingredients

- 1 cup of raw oats, preferably gluten-free (the best would be: sprouted, or: Scottish, as well as rolled oats, oat grouts—make sure that they are unprocessed and truly raw).
- 1 cup of raw almond milk or raw oat milk
- 1 cup of blueberries
- 1 cup of strawberries, cut in halves
- A few raisins
- Juice of1 lemon
- 1 tablespoon of coconut oil
- 1tablespoon of cinnamon
- 1 tablespoon of cocoa powder (raw, of course)

Instructions

1. Soak the oats for a few hours (or, you can just soak them overnight) in 1 cup of vegan milk with tiny bit of water if you wish. Add 1 tablespoon of cinnamon. It will give it a nice and sweet taste, and if you are struggling to give up sugar, it will serve you as a natural and healthy replacement.
2. In a bowl, mix the soaked oats with the blueberries and strawberries (cut them in halves or in slices, whatever suits your visual preferences).
3. Add a few raisins and 1 tablespoon of coconut oil.
4. Finally, add lemon juice (of 1 lemon) to make it more alkaline.
5. Sprinkle over some cocoa powder. I also like to add half a teaspoon of powdered spiruline, chlorella, or alfalfa powder (this one is really good for your skin and hair!).

Serve chilled or, if you are really hungry—immediately! Have a nice and energetic day!

RECIPE#18 Raw Peppers

This is one of those recipes that is really visually appealing. Test it, make some for your family and friends, and I can guarantee that it will be gone in less than a few minutes!

This is a great recipe for the summer, and it is really easy to prepare. It can also serve as a healthy aperitif.

Serves-2

Ingredients

- 2 red peppers
- ¼ cup of chia seeds
- 4 pineapple slices
- 1 onion
- 1 cup of radishes
- 1 tablespoon of curry powder
- 1 tablespoon of coconut oil
- ½ cup of coconut milk
- 1 avocado
- 2 garlic cloves
- 1 cucumber
- 4 tomatoes
- 1 teaspoon of rosemary herb
- Himalaya salt (optional)
- Pepper

Instructions

1. Wash the peppers, cut into halves, and remove the seeds. Set aside. Optional- you may smear the insides with some coconut oil.
2. Wash and peel the tomatoes and avocado (remove the pit).
3. In a blender, mix the tomatoes, avocado, coconut oil, coconut milk, and 2 garlic cloves (remove the peel). Blend and add 1 tablespoon of curry powder.
4. Wash and peel the cucumber and onion. Mince them. Wash and slice the radishes and pineapple slices.
5. In a bowl, mix the ingredients from step 4. With the blended ingredients from the step 3. Mix in some rosemary herb and chia seeds.
6. Season with some pepper and Himalaya salt.
7. Equally distribute the filling on each red pepper half. Squeeze in some lemon juice. So yummy!

Enjoy!

***Variations and Tips (not for hardcore raw-foodists)

Raw foods can be easily combined with other diets and they will always bring some healthy balance and more nutrients. It's up to you if you want to keep it vegan, raw or mix it and adapt it according to your lifestyle. I am just giving you some cooking ideas that you and your family can enjoy!

I have also tried this recipe with some grains such as quinoa, millet, and brown rice. Not raw foody, but vegan and a great source of good carbohydrates.

RECIPE#19 Spicy Beetroot Salad

I used to hate beetroots, now I love them. I think it all comes down to experimenting with different tastes and combinations. This is what the raw food art is all about.

Serves-2

Ingredients

- 4 raw beetroots
- 1 cup of radishes
- 1 onion
- 1 garlic clove
- 1 pinch of chili powder
- 2 apples
- 1 cucumber
- Olive oil
- Juice of 1 lemon

Instructions

1. Wash, peel and slice the beets (make them really thin slices).
2. Wash and slice the radishes.
3. Wash, peel and slice the cucumber and apples.
4. Wash, peel and mince the garlic and onions.
5. Mix all the ingredients in a bowl, add 1 pinch of chili powder, fresh lemon juice and olive oil.

Serve immediately!

RECIPE#20 Anti-cellulite

If you suffer from cellulite, water retention or slow digestion, this recipe can help you. Make sure you have this salad at least 3 times a week. Feel free to experiment and make different variations so as not to get bored with it. You can also blend the ingredients.

Serves-2,3

Ingredients

- 1 pineapple
- 2 apples
- 1 cucumber
- 1 cup of blueberries
- ½ cup of coconut milk
- Juice of 1 lemon

Instructions

1. Wash and peel the pineapple. Cut it into little cubes.
2. Wash and peel the apples and cucumber. Cut them in halves and slice them.
3. In a bowl, mix with blueberries (remember to wash them), some coconut milk and fresh lemon juice.
4. Garnish with a slice of lemon or lime.

It's refreshing, re-mineralizing and really good for your microcirculation.

Pineapple and pineapple extracts are used by many naturopaths as a natural supplement in weight loss, fat burn and anti-cellulite diets.

RECIPE#21 Broccoli Salad

I know people who eat raw broccoli; however I prefer to steam it or cook it a bit in low temperatures. The raw food guideline says that you should eat foods that were uncooked and unprocessed, or slightly cooked (no more than 30-40 Celsius degrees). It's totally up to you how you want to have this recipe. I am showing you my way!

Serves-2

Ingredients

- 2 cups of broccoli crowns (chopped into small pieces)
- Half cup of raisins
- 1 cup of baby spinach
- 2 garlic cloves
- Half onion
- 1 apple
- 2 tablespoons of vegan maple syrup
- 2 tablespoons of olive oil
- Raw cashews powder
- Juice of one lemon

Instructions

1. If you don't want your broccoli 100% raw, steam it or cook it. I like to cook it in 20 degrees filtered water (for about 15 minutes). I actually use this water for soups and creams, if there are any nutrients that did not want to stay in a broccoli, I will still get them! Makes sense, right?
2. In the meantime, wash and chop the spinach and apples. The same with onions.

3. Grate garlic cloves and in a little cup, mix it with olive oil and maple syrup. You may add some Himalaya salt.
4. Mix broccolis with raisins, onions and apples. Spread on the salsa. Sprinkle over some cashews powder as if it was "normal" cheese.
5. Sprinkle over some fresh lemon juice (Alkalinity!).

OPTIONAL: if you feel like cheating on the raw foods diet, you may add some organic mustard to spice up your broccoli salad. I do it from time to time. Like, I said, I don't do the raw foods full-time.

RECIPE#22 Mozarella Tomato Salad with no Mozarella!

This recipe is a vegan version of "tomato mozzarella".

Serves-2

Ingredients

- 6 raw tomatoes
- 2 garlic cloves
- Half cup of fresh basil leaves
- ¼ cup of chopped chive
- Pinch of black pepper
- Himalaya salt
- Olive Oil
- Balsamic Vinegar (raw, organic)
- 1 big avocado
- Rosemary herb

Instructions

1. Wash and slice the tomatoes, place them on a plate.
2. Wash, peel, pit and slice the avocado, place together with the tomatoes, just as if it was mozzarella cheese.
3. Equally distribute some fresh basil leaves and chive.
4. Sprinkle over some rosemary herb, balsamic vinegar, some pepper, salt and olive oil (I usually use 2 tablespoons of each). Serve chilled!

RECIPE#23 Cauliflower Salad with Thai Twist

This recipe has the same philosophy as the one with broccoli. It's OK to steam or cook your cauliflower a bit- for most people it means- easier digestion. I believe that there is no need to be a radical raw foods martyr, even if you want to do it full-time, the rule is clear- as long as the foods have been cooked in a temperature not higher than 30-40 degrees (Celsius) it is still considered pretty raw.

Even if that concerns you, you can still create some raw balance by eating this pre-cooked or steamed veggie with some raw dressing. I love the creativity that the raw foods or alkaline diet foods have as far as salads are concerned. A yummy dressing can make it a real pleasure for your taste buds. I think it's also a fantastic idea to gradually get used to making your own salad dressing and experimenting with different oils, herbs, and spices. The modern world is full of chemically processed condiments that, in my opinion, should be avoided at all costs. Regardless of which diets you have chosen to follow or how many calories are on the label. What I am more concerned about is the list of crazy ingredients that are hard or impossible to pronounce; for me, it's a big "no"!

Back to our cauliflower, you can also pre-soak it in some warm water with a bit of spices to give it a nice flavor (I like to put some chili, powdered garlic, and curry). It's up to you, choose your own way, but, of course, try to keep it as raw as possible.

Serves-2

Ingredients

- 2 cups of pre-steamed, pre-cooked, or (if you wish) raw cauliflower crowns chopped in small pieces (the visual part is up to you, whatever you find more appealing)
- 1 cup of alfalfa sprouts
- A few kale leaves
- Juice of 1 lemon

For the dressing:

- 4 tablespoons of raw tahini
- Juice of 1 lime
- 1/2cup of raw almond powder
- 3 tablespoons of tamari
- 2 tablespoons of vegan maple syrup
- 2 garlic cloves
- Ginger (more or less the same amount as garlic)

Instructions

1. In a bowl, mix chopped cauliflower crowns with a few kale leaves and alfalfa sprouts.
2. Sprinkle over some fresh lemon juice.
3. Prepare the dressing: blend all the ingredients until smooth.
4. Mix with the cauliflower salad.

Who said cauliflower can't be tasty...?

RECIPE#24 Alfalfa Green Alkaline Salad

Alfalfa is extremely alkalizing, just like other green vegetables. If you feel like you cannot focus, have low energy levels, and are looking for a natural beauty treatment as well, you should definitely add some green foods to your diet. I am not saying that these are some magical cure for everything (unfortunately, the whole green foods idea is getting a little bit overhyped these days), but one thing is sure, they won't hurt and they will be a great addition to whatever diet you have chosen to do!

Serves-2

Ingredients

- 1 cup of alfalfa sprouts
- ¼ cup of chopped chives
- 2 cups of baby spinach
- ½ cup of almonds
- Pinch of curry powder (I like this oriental taste in all my salads!)
- 1 avocado
- Juice of 1 lime
- ¼ cup of fresh basil
- A few mint leaves to garnish
- 2 tablespoons of olive oil
- A few raisins

Instructions

1. Wash the alfalfa sprouts and spinach, chop finely (or the way you wish to see them on your plate).

2. Wash, peel, and pit the avocado. Slice and mix with alfalfa and spinach.
3. In a bowl, mix with chives, almonds, minced garlic, and basil.
4. Sprinkle over the lime juice, a few raisins and olive oil.
5. Garnish with some fresh mint.

Serve immediately!

Enjoy!

RECIPE#25 Raw Paleo Inspired Dessert

When hearing the word "Paleo", many people immediately think about massive amounts of meat. However, Paleo desserts are a different story. And even though the Paleo diet is totally different than a vegan diet (I think it's obvious), Paleo desserts and vegan- raw desserts very often overlap. The reason is simple, the rules are the same: no processed foods, only fresh fruits and vegetables and lots of creativity...Anyway, this recipe is really kids' friendly!

Serves-2,3

Ingredients

- 2 bananas
- 2 avocados
- 2 cups of raw almond milk
- 2 tablespoons of stevia
- 1 tablespoon of coconut oil
- 4 tablespoons of raw cocoa powder

Instructions

1. Wash and peel the avocado (remove the oil of course) and bananas. Slice and place in a blender.
2. Mix with other ingredients and blend until smooth.
3. Place the raw, yummy cream in a fridge for 30 minutes- 1 hour to serve it cold.
4. Serve with a few pinches of cinnamon.

My suggestion: add one teaspoon of chlorella or spiruline powder to make it even more energizing. I am now using alfalfa sprouts powder, and I love it in my smoothies of all kinds (the taste of chlorella and spiruline can be too much for some people; I am used to it, but I know that many people would prefer alfalfa. I really recommend it as a natural supplement. It's also great for your skin and hair).

RECIPE#26 Zucchini Asparagus Greek Salad

I love zucchini! I first though that I would not be able to have them on the raw food diet. I mean, eating them 100% raw did not seem like a good idea to me. I always used to make different zucchini dishes with my oven, but then I realized that the raw food diet allows you to use lower temperatures for food preparation.

Remember that the raw dressing will make up for the possible loss of nutrients during the cooking process.

Serves:2

Ingredients

- 2 big zucchini
- About 10 asparagus
- 1 cup of black olives, pitted
- 1 cup of green olives, pitted
- 2 tablespoons of sesame seeds
- 2 tablespoons of olive oil
- Juice of 1 lemon
- 1 avocado, peeled and pitted
- 2 garlic cloves
- Rosemary herb
- Himalaya salt
- Pinch of curry powder
- Black pepper

Instructions

1. Wash and slice zucchini and cook or steam slightly in a temperature that does not exceed 30-40 degrees Celsius. 10 minutes should be enough.
2. Do the same with asparagus- you can even steam/ cook them together
3. In the meantime mince the garlic and blend with lemon juice, olive oil, and avocado. Add some rosemary, Himalaya salt, curry and pepper to taste.
4. Dry the zucchini and asparagus; chop them the way you wish to see them on your plate and mix with olives. Sprinkle over the mix from step 3.

So delicious and refreshing!

RECIPE#27 Before Workout Smoothie

I know that many people can't even imagine eating broccoli and kale. They just hate the taste. If you find it hard to force yourself to eat broccoli and kale, you should try this smoothie. It will help you enjoy the benefits of those vegetables and the sweet taste. Is it possible? Yes, just follow me!

This is a fantastic before or after workout smoothie. It's always better to fuel your body before you hit the gym, and the liquid diet facilitates digestion so your body will have more energy to focus on burning fat and building on muscles.

Don't go to the gym hungry, but also avoid overeating. Choose a smoothie; this one is really one of the best I can recommend!

Serves:1

Ingredients

- 2 bananas
- Half cup of coconut milk
- Half cup of coconut water (it's great after a workout by the way!)
- 1 cup of broccoli crowns
- A few leaves of kale
- 1 teaspoon of cinnamon
- A few raisins and dates (optional)
- 1 kiwi (you also want some natural sources of vitamin C!).

Instructions

1. Wash and peel the bananas and kiwi.

2. In a blender, mix with broccoli crowns and kale leaves; add coconut milk and coconut water and a few raisins and dates if you want to make it sweet.
3. Blend until smooth.
4. Sprinkle over some cinnamon.

OPTIONAL: if you have some powdered alfalfa natural supplement you may add it to your smoothie to alkalinize it. If not, why not? This is just a quick alkaline tip that everyone can benefit from!

RECIPE#28 Refreshing Choco Smoothie!

I used to think that there are no sweets on the raw food diet. I was wrong—you are allowed to give yourself some healthy pleasure every now and then. I love experimenting with smoothies and combining different tastes. I think that this recipe is an excellent example of how you can combine sour with sweet and achieve perfect balance! Remember, smoothies are not something you should feel guilty drinking. They are nutritious and provide your body with more energy to function at its optimal levels. In my opinion, when you eat clean, alkaline, raw foods on a regular basis (70% is already and excellent result), there is no need to be obsessed about counting calories. This is also a really kid friendly smoothie. I have noticed that very few kids like grapefruits or lemons, and I can't blame them for that. I would be a bit worried about a kid who loves lemons and hates chocolate, ha-ha! When I was a kid, my dad would make me eat grapefruit, but he would always slice them as if they were bread and smear them with some syrup or cane sugar, and sprinkle over some cinnamon, I am very grateful to my parents that they thought me to eat healthy from an early age.

Serves: 2-3

Ingredients

- Juice of 2 oranges
- Juice of 2 lemons
- Juice of 2 oranges
- 4 tablespoons of raw cocoa powder
- 2 kiwis

- 1 cup of coconut milk or almond milk
- 2 tablespoons of sesame powder

Instructions

1. Squeeze some the lemons, oranges and grapefruits.
2. In a blender, mix the citrus mix juice with cocoa powder, sesame powder, peeled kiwis and coconut milk.
3. Blend until smooth.
4. Garnish with some fresh mint leaves and a few sprinkles of cinnamon.

OPTIONAL

Depending on your blender, you may also skip step 1 and just blend all the ingredients together. I prefer to squeeze the juice first; it's also fault of my rather "mediocre" blender (I hope to be able to invest in a better one soon!).

My reflection: just like there are some people who can't stand the sour taste of certain fruits, some people hate it when it's too sweet, and they can even get headaches or nausea after eating something sweet. If you fall into the second category, I would definitely recommend this smoothie. The way the tasty balance is achieved here is just amazing!

RECIPE#29 Oriental Aphrodisiac Smoothie

I am sure you have heard of maca powder and its stimulating and aphrodisiac properties. To be honest, I don't really believe in "small aphrodisiac cures". I think that the only one that exists and works in the long-run is healthy lifestyle. Here is another reason why you want to eat more raw foods. People who eat at least 60-70% of raw, natural, unprocessed, and alkaline foods have it much easier to lose weight in a natural way, enjoy more energy levels, confidence, and of course, a sexy body. What more can you ask for?

This recipe contains some amazing oriental spices that are great for the senses. If you want to have beautiful, healthy skin or have it difficult to get tanned, then you should add more carrots into your diet, they contain beta-carotene and also help protect your skin from sunburn.

Overall, this raw smoothie is an excellent combination of raw foods, spices, and of course, the magical maca powder! Whether it is an aphrodisiac or not (maybe it is being a bit overhyped these days), it is rich in vitamin C, iron, and calcium and helps maintain a healthy alkaline balanced in our body. So it can't hurt!

Serves: 2

Ingredients

- 6 carrots
- 1 banana
- 1 cup of coconut water
- Half cup of coconut milk

- 2 tablespoons of cinnamon
- 2 tablespoons of maca powder
- 2 tablespoons of vegan maple syrup
- 1 pinch of cloves herb
- 2 tablespoons of mixed ginger
- 1 tablespoon of nutmeg

Instructions

1. Wash and peel the carrots and banana. Cut into smaller pieces you're your blender will accept.
2. Mix with coconut milk and coconut water and add the ginger and spices. Blend until smooth.
3. Add some maple syrup to taste + maca powder. Stir for about 2 minutes.

Serve immediately! Garnish with a slice of lime.

Enjoy!

RECIPE#30 Creamy Wakame Smoothie

Hold on, I know what you are thinking, how can a seaweed such as wakame be tasty and creamy? What is she talking about?

Ok, first let me tell you what alga wakame provides you with (yes I know that when served raw, its taste might be far from pleasurable!), it is rich in:

- Vitamin A
- Vitamin C
- Vitamin E
- Vitamin K
- Niacin (excellent for your hair and skin!)
- Phosphorus
- Calcium
- Magnesium (one of the most alkaline minerals!)
- Iron (this is why wakame is an excellent solution for vegans and vegetarians!)
- Manganese
- Riboflavin
- Panthothenic Acid

So many nutrients just in one seaweed, yes!

For me, the best and the easiest way to make sure that I function at the optimal levels and can lead my active lifestyle the way I want to, is to use foods such as wakame in my diet. This is why I don't need any artificial and expensive supplements.

Do I like the way alga wakame tastes raw? To be honest, there are much more pleasurable eating sensations that my taste buds go for, but I learned how to take wakame in my smoothies (sweet) or in my salads (spicy and tasty). Now, I buy it on a regular basis. I really recommend you add alga wakame to your diet. Don't be put off by its taste; you can change it with this amazing smoothie!

Serves: 2

Ingredients

- About 5 square centimeters of dry alga wakame
- 1 cup of coconut milk
- 1 cup of rice milk or almond milk
- 2 teaspoons of cinnamon
- 4 peaches (pitted)
- 1 banana
- 1 kiwi

Instructions

1. Soak alga wakame in cold water (for about 15 minutes)
2. In the meantime, wash and pit the peaches. Wash and peel the banana and kiwi. Cut into small pieces.
3. In a blender, mix the fruits with the coconut milk and the rice milk, add wakame and blend until smooth.
4. Add cinnamon powder and stir energetically.

Serve with some ice cubes and a slice of lemon!

Enjoy, and think of all the benefits that wakame provides you with!

Wakame may seem expensive at first, but when you buy it, you will see that it will last a very long time. This is because when you soak it, it doubles and even triples in size.

RECIPE#31 Lovely Apple Dip!

If you feel like having something sweet and incredibly healthy, here is my plan for you. Like I said earlier, you can also enjoy some healthy sweets on the raw food diets!

Serves: 3,4

Ingredients

For the dip:

- 4 apples, peeled
- 4 pears, peeled
- 2 tablespoons of cinnamon
- 1 teaspoon of nutmeg
- 2 tablespoons of vegan maple syrup
- Juice of 1 lemon
- 1 cup of coconut milk
- 1 tablespoon of coconut oil

For the snack:

- 4 carrots
- 1 tablespoon of maple syrup
- Almond powder

Instructions

1. Wash and peel the apples and pears. Cut into smaller pieces that your blender will like.
2. In a blender, mix with coconut milk, lemon juice, nutmeg, cinnamon, honey and coconut oil. Blend until smooth. Set aside in a fridge.

3. In the meantime, wash and peel the carrots. Smear them with some maple syrup, and sprinkle over some almond powder.
4. Serve with the apple dip. Eat to your health!

Enjoy!

RECIPE#32 Raw Italian Food

Even if you decide to go for raw and vegan options, you can still enjoy your favorite "comfort" flavors and tastes.

Check out this recipe; it's very easy to make and can satisfy your "Italian" tooth.

Serves: 2

Ingredients

- 4 zucchini (for the raw noodles)
- 2 cups of cherry tomatoes
- 2 cloves of garlic
- 1 tablespoon of fresh oregano
- 1 tablespoon of fresh basin
- 2 tablespoons of olive oil
- 1 onion
- Pinch of Himalaya salt

Instructions

1. Use spiralizer to create zucchini noodles. If you wish, you may also steam your noodles slightly before serving.
2. Now it's time to prepare our raw Italian salsa: in a blender, mix the cherry tomatoes with the Italian herbs, olive oil, garlic, and onion. Blend until smooth. You may want to use a sieve so get rid of tomato skin.
3. Taste your salsa to check whether you need to use more pepper to salt.
4. Serve the raw salsa with your noodles.
5. Optional: sprinkle over some powdered almonds or cashnuts. Raw vegan world is so creative!

6. Sprinkle over some fresh lemon juice.
7. Enjoy, I do!

RECIPE#33 Raw Thai Dip

This is a delicious, raw Thai dip that you can serve with veggies (cucumbers, carrots, zucchinis) to give them more taste. I also like it as a healthy snack with peppers for example.

Serves: 2

Ingredients

- 1 cup of almond butter (make sure it is raw and unprocessed)
- 1 cup of fresh orange juice
- 2 tablespoons of minced ginger
- Soy sauce (about 2 tablespoons)
- 2 garlic cloves, minced
- 2 tablespoons of vegan maple syrup
- 1 pinch of cayenne pepper

Instructions

1. Mix all the ingredients in a blender.

2. Add some Himalaya salt and cayenne pepper to taste.

3. Serve with some nice and fresh raw veggies of your choice. I also like it with apples.

RECIPE#34 Nori Wraps

Nori is a famous sushi ingredient, but the truth is that it can be used for a whole range of wraps and rolls.

Serves: 1-2

Ingredients

- 4 sheets of alga nori
- 1 avocado
- 2 garlic cloves
- 1 cucumber
- 2 carrots
- 1 apple
- 1 onion
- 4 tomatoes
- A few radishes
- Coconut oil
- 1 lemon

Instructions

1. Wash and peel the ingredients.
2. Chop them finely. Mince garlic and onion and add to the mix.
3. Smear some coconut oil on each nori sheet and add the filling. Form wraps.
4. Sprinkle over some lemon juice.

Enjoy!

RECIPE#35 Raw Toasts with Raw Nutella

The raw food diet is about replacing and creating and always looking for healthier alternatives. I love chocolate and nutella. I used to think that nutella is something that you could only eat on toast (yummy but too many calories). The raw food diet made me realize that other, healthier options exist...

This is an excellent and energetic snack where a perfect balance is found!

Serves:2

Ingredients

- 2 big red or green apples (I like acidic apples with this recipe)
- Half cup of almond milk
- Half cup of ground hazelnuts
- 4 tablespoons of cocoa powder
- Cinnamon powder

Instructions

1. Wash and slice the apples. They will be our version of toast!
2. In a blender, mix almond milk with ground hazelnuts and cocoa powder. This will be our raw and healthy unprocessed and sugar free nutella.
3. Smear the nutella on each apple slice and sprinkle over some cinnamon. So delicious!

OPTION B:

You can also make your own almond butter. Just soak 1 cup of almonds overnight, add some cinnamon to taste. Then, blend them with some coconut milk and coconut oil. Experiment so as to achieve your desired texture. You can have it with apples, pearls, pineapples, or kiwis!

RECIPE#36 Parsley Soup

When I was a kid, my dad introduced me to eating parsley raw. Yes!

You heard me right- raw as a snack. He would always tell me that parsley is an excellent source of Vitamin A and is good for me eyes. He would always sprinkle over some parsley on my sandwich or soup. Now, if you can't imagine eating it raw as a rabbit or little Marta, haha, try this delicious parsley soup recipe!

Serves-2

Ingredients

- 1 cup of parsley
- 1 onion, peeled and chopped
- 6 ripe tomatoes, peeled
- Half cup raw pistachios (remove shells)
- Half teaspoon curry powder
- 1 pinch of Himalaya salt
- A few basil leaves
- A few mint leaves (it will add an amazing taste to this soup!)
- 2cups of water
- 1 cup of coconut milk
- 2 tablespoons of olive oil

Instructions

1. In a blender, mix the tomatoes, onion, parsley, water, and coconut milk. Add some coconut oil, curry, mint, and basil leaves, and blend until smooth.
2. Cool it down in a fridge, and serve with some raw pistachios. Add some salt and pepper to taste.
3. Garnish with mint leaves!
4. Enjoy!

RECIPE#37 Pumpkin Almost Raw Soup

I love raw soups and creams! Pumpkin is great for your skin as it is loaded with natural beta-carotene, niacin, Thiamin, and Vitamin E. Apart from its anti-aging properties, it is also a great source of iron, Magnesium, Phosphorus, Vitamin A, Vitamin C, and dietary fiber. Switching to raw foods, or making them at least 50% of your diet, will nourish your body in a natural way, and there will be no need to reach out to artificial vitamin supplements. You will be experiencing amazing energy levels all the time.

The reason why I called this recipe "almost raw" is that we will be soaking pumpkin in warm water (no more than 30 degrees Celsius, so that it still sticks to the raw food rules).

Serves:2

Ingredients

- 1 small pumpkin, peeled
- 2 carrots
- 1 cucumber
- 2 tablespoons of coconut oil
- 1 garlic clove
- 1 pinch of chili powder
- Half teaspoon of curry powder
- Half cup of water
- Half cup of almond milk or coconut milk
- Pinch of Himalaya salt

Instructions

1. After peeling the pumpkin, chop it into small pieces, and let it soak in warm water for about 15 minutes.

Make sure that the water's temperature does not exceed 30 degrees Celsius.

2. In the meantime, wash and peel the carrots, cucumber, and garlic clove. Cut into smaller pieces, and in a blender, mix with some water, almond or coconut milk. Blend until smooth and add the pumpkin.

3. Add some coconut oil for better taste and more nutritional value (good fats!), and season with some curry powder, chili powder, and salt. If you find the texture too thin, add some crashed almonds or other nuts, if you find it too thick, add some water or coconut milk.

4. Serve chilled. Garnish with some mint leaves, enjoy!

RECIPE#38 "Going Nuts" Mix for Students

When I was a kid, my grandparents would always tell me that eating nuts would help me study better and faster. Maybe it was a placebo effect, but I would always have a cup of raw nuts when doing my homework or studying for an exam, and I felt like I could concentrate much better. I also love nuts before my workouts.

Nuts are rich in vitamins, minerals, protein, and omega-3 fatty acids and are an excellent addition to a raw food diet.

Serves-1

Ingredients

- 1 cup of hazelnut milk (if you are concerned about calorie intake, use coconut water or aloe vera water instead)
- 1 tablespoon of almonds
- 1 tablespoon of chia seeds
- 1 tablespoon of cashew nuts
- Half cup of blueberries or raspberries
- Half avocado, peeled and pitted

Instructions

Mix all the ingredients in a bowl, and enjoy your super quick and natural snack!

OPTIONAL: if you are a student and are feeling mentally exhausted during your exams, add one teaspoon of soy lecithin.

RECIPE#39 Mango-Banana Dairy Free Ice-Cream

Here comes one of my favorite summer refreshments!

Try it yourself...

Serves-2

Ingredients

- 2 bananas
- 1 big mango
- ¼ cup of mint leaves
- 2 cups of almond milk
- 1 tablespoons of coconut oil
- 1 tablespoon of natural vanilla extract (optional)

+ half banana and a few mint leaves to garnish

Instructions

1. Wash and peel the bananas and mango, remove pit from mango. Cut into smaller pieces.
2. In a blender, mix them with almond milk and fresh mint leaves. Add 2 tablespoons of coconut oil, and blend until smooth.
3. Distribute into 2 little cups or bowl and place in a freezer for a few hours.
4. Garnish with some banana slices and fresh mint leaves. I like to squeeze in some fresh lime juice on it!

Why would you crave some unhealthy ice-cream filled with artificial ingredients and empty calories when you have this amazingly delicious raw food ice-cream recipe?

RECIPE#40 Delicious Raw Salsa

Salsas are what makes the raw foods exciting and fun.

You can use raw salsas with some raw veggies or salads, or if you decide to do the raw foods part-time, you can also mix it with some cooked foods to at least try to make up for some lost nutrients.

Ingredients

- 8 ripe tomatoes
- 3 cloves of garlic
- 1 cup of tomato juice (just blend a few tomatoes and sprinkle over some olive oil)
- 1 tablespoon of fresh, chopped cilantro
- 1 Serrano pepper
- 1/2 teaspoon ground cumin
- Half teaspoon of vegan maple syrup
- 3 green onions
- Juice of 1 lemon

Instructions

1. Wash and peel the tomatoes, garlic, and onions. Chop into smaller pieces.

2. Wash and chop the peppers.

3. In a blender, mix all the ingredients with some fresh tomato juice and lime juice. Add the spices. Blend until smooth.

4. Garnish with some basil leaves. Serve with some cucumber or carrot sticks.

Enjoy!

RECIPE#41 Amazingly Refreshing Cucumber Soup

Here comes another refreshing, raw food, summer recipe!

Serves-2

Ingredients

- 2 teaspoons olive oil
- 5 cucumbers, peeled and chopped
- 3 cloves of garlic
- 2 onions, diced
- 1 cup of fresh tomato juice (just blend a few tomatoes to make your own)
- 1/4 cup chopped fresh dill
- Black pepper to taste
- 1 cup almond milk
- Juice of 2 limes
- Himalaya salt

Instructions

1. In a blender, mix the cucumbers with fresh tomato juice, lime juice, and almond milk.
2. Add onions, garlic and blend.
3. Add a pinch of Himalaya salt, black pepper, and fresh dill.
4. Serve immediately!

Enjoy!

RECIPE#42 Refreshing Colors Salad

Salads are not only the pleasure to our taste buds, but also to our eyes!

Having some kiwi in this massive salad makes it a bit exotic and gives it a nice flavor!

Serves-4
Ingredients
- Half of iceberg lettuce
- 1 green pepper
- 1 red pepper
- 1 orange/yellow pepper
- 4 carrots
- 2 cucumbers
- 1 cup of radishes
- 2 tomatoes
- 1 cup of almonds
- 1 red onion
- ¼ cup of chopped chives
- 2 kiwis
- White asparagus, slightly steamed
- Olive oil
- Juice of 1 lemon
- Black pepper
- Soy sauce
- Oregano

Instructions

1. Wash and peel the veggies and kiwis.
2. Mince the onion, slice carrots, iceberg lettuce, peppers, cucumbers, radishes, tomatoes, kiwis and asparagus.
3. Mix all the ingredients in a bowl and some almonds and sprinkle over some fresh lemon juice, soy sauce and olive oil. Add some oregano to taste.

So fresh, tasty and alkalizing!

RECIPE#43 Watermelon Gazpacho

Who said that only tomatoes and cucumbers have a monopoly on the gazpacho recipes?

Try this recipe and discover another version of gazpacho; it is extremely refreshing!

Serves-2,3

Ingredients

- 8 ripe tomatoes
- 1 watermelon (remove the skin)
- 2 onions (peeled and sliced)
- 2 garlic cloves
- 1 tablespoon olive oil
- 2 tablespoons vinegar
- 1 pinch of salt
- Optional: 1 cup of filtered water or aloe vera water

Instructions

1. Wash and peel the tomatoes, onions and garlic.
2. In a blender, mix tomatoes, garlic, and onions with watermelon chunks.
3. Add some olive oil, and if you want it to be smoother, add some filtered water or aloe vera water.
4. Add some salt and pepper to taste.
5. Serve chilled!

An excellent dish for hot summer days!

RECIPE#44 Raw Carrots Cream

This is another simple and creamy recipe that is packed with beta-carotene for amazingly healthy skin!

Serves-2

Ingredients

- 6 carrots
- (Optional and not raw) 1 sweet potato, slightly boiled
- 1 onion
- 2 garlic cloves
- 1 bay leaf
- 2 cups water (you can also experiment and use some aloe vera water or coconut water, these are packed with nutrients)
- 2 tablespoons olive oil
- Salt and pepper
- Some chili powder if you like it spicy
- 1 cup of natural vegan yogurt (can be GMO free soy yoghurt, almond yoghurt or any non-dairy yoghurt of your choice. If you are not vegan, you can also try some Greek yoghurt- it's creamy and delicious)

Instructions

1. Wash and peel the carrots, onions, and garlic. Chop into smaller pieces that your blender can handle.
2. In a blender, mix the ingredients with some water and blend until smooth.
3. Add some yogurt, olive oil, salt, and spices.
4. Garnish with bay leaf.
5. Serve natural or chilled. Enjoy!

RECIPE#45 Energizing Chia Seeds Water

I am a strong believer in the alkaline diet, so I can never stress enough the importance of hydration. I know that some of you may not like our all good and boring H2O. This is a recipe for alkaline and raw, super healthy lemonade. No more soft drinks or sodas! Make it natural and healthy. I like to have 2 glasses of this amazing drink first thing in the morning to make sure I am full of energy to start my day.

Ingredients for 4-5 glasses (cups)

- 1 tablespoon chia seeds (soaked in water for a few hours)
- Fresh juice of 2 lemons
- Fresh juice of 3 limes
- 3 tablespoons of vegan maple syrup
- 1 liter of filtered water
- Optional: 1 cup of aloe vera water or coconut water
- A few leaves of fresh mint
- 2 mandarins

Instructions

1. Blend all the ingredients except for mandarins and mint leaves and stir energetically.
2. Put the lemon water in a big jar. Throw in a few mint leaves and mandarin chunks. These will give your water more flavors. Fruit infused water is a big thing these days. While it may be a little bit overhyped, it is certainly really healthy. Try it yourself!
3. Add some ice cubes if you wish. Your natural alkaline drink is ready!

RECIPE#46 Hunger Killing Garlic Soup

This soup has some natural antibiotic properties and it is an excellent natural remedy that strengthens your immune system.

Serves-2

Ingredients

- OPTIONAL(it does not really form part of raw foods)- half cup of integral, gluten-free bread crumbs
- Half cup of raw almonds powder
- 4 cloves of garlic
- 1 cucumber
- 2 cups of filtered water
- 2 tablespoons of olive oil
- 1 dash of balsamic vinegar
- Himalaya salt
- Black pepper

Instructions

1. Wash and peel the cucumber and garlic cloves. Slice and put in a blender.

2. Add some filtered water, raw almond powder, olive oil, and balsamic vinegar. Blend until smooth.

3. Season with some salt and black pepper to taste. I like to sprinkle over some fresh lime or lemon juice.

So delicious and healthy!

RECIPE#47 Raw Greek Tzaziki with Seeds

This is a quick and refreshing dip to serve when you have some friends over. I like it with some olives, radishes, and peppers. Don't forget an occasional glass of organic wine!

If you don't do the raw foods diet full-time, I also recommend you try it with some cus-cus, brown rice, or boiled potatoes. There are so many options out there to combine raw uncooked foods with other diets and way of eating!

Serves-2

Ingredients

- 3 cucumbers
- 1 garlic clove, peeled
- Two natural soy yogurts or other vegan yogurts(sugar free!)
- 1 teaspoon dill
- 1 tablespoon olive oil
- Salt and pepper to taste
- Few drops of lemon
- 2 tablespoons of sesame seeds (better ground)

Instructions

1. Wash and peel the cucumbers.
2. In a blender, mix with garlic, yogurt, dill, olive oil, salt, pepper, sesame seeds and fresh lemon juice.
3. Blend until smooth.
4. Garnish with some fresh lime slices or mint leaves.

RECIPE#48 Catalan Carrot "Alioli"

This recipe is inspired by the traditional Spanish-Catalan "alioli", which is a garlic cream that can really spice up your meals.

Serves-2

Ingredients

- 2 carrots
- 6 garlic cloves (peeled)
- Himalaya salt
- Fresh juice of 1 lemon
- Olive oil (4 tablespoons)

Instructions

1. Wash and peel the carrots.

2. In a blender, mix with garlic cloves, olive oil, lemon juice, and Himalaya salt.

3. Blend until smooth.

This dip will make all your raw foods taste amazing! Try it with some broccoli... So yummy!

MY TIP: It also tastes amazing with tofu, rice and raw or even cooked veggies. As you have probably noticed, I am very open-minded when it comes to different diets, and I am happy to provide you with my recipes and tips, so that you can adapt them to your own lifestyle. Like I said in the introduction, even if you are neither a vegan nor a vegetarian, you can still do raw foods part-time. Just try to incorporate them as much as you can. Natural salsas and dips are full of nutrients and are a great alternative to give up all those processed condiments that are extremely acidic.

RECIPE#49 Your Own Organic Raw Almond Milk

I used to buy almond milk, but ever since I discovered how easy it is to make my own, I just went for it. That way I am sure that my almond milk is pure and organic, and I also save lots of money. As you may have noticed, I use almond milk quite a lot, in fact, it is my favorite vegan milk.

Ingredients for 4 cups approx
- 1 cup raw peeled almonds (200 gr. Approx.)
- 1 liter of water
- A few dates (pitted), a banana and 2 tablespoons of vegan maple syrup if you like it sweet. I encourage you to try different options and see what works for you.

Instructions
1. Soak almonds in 1 liter of filtered water for at least 2 hours. I usually leave it overnight.
2. Blend the soaked almonds (use the same water you used for soaking them) with a banana, dates, and syrup. Make sure it's all smoothed.
3. Use a filter or a sieve to separate the liquid from soaked almond "mass".

*I suggest you use the almond "mass" for natural butters (just mix it with some cocoa powder and coconut oil and milk). You can also use it for vegetable creams and soups to give them more consistency.

As for the almond milk--serve chilled with some ice cubes and sprinkle over some cinnamon or/and cocoa powder. Enjoy!

RECIPE#50 Spanish Alkalizing Granizado

Here comes another refreshing summer drink!
It takes about half an hour to prepare it.

Serves: 4-5
Ingredients
- 8 big lemons
- A few tablespoons of raw organic vegan maple syrup
- 1 liter of water

Instructions
1. Squeeze the lemons. Mix the fresh orange juice with water.
2. Add some vegan maple syrup and stir energetically.
3. Pour into small cups or dessert bowls.
4. Put in a freezer for about 30 minutes. We want some natural ice cubes in there but don't want it to become totally frozen (unless you want a watery ice-cream).
5. Garnish with slice of lemon or fresh mint leaves.

OPTIONAL
I like to use alga agar-agar with this recipe. I take about 1 cup of dried agar-agar and soak it in filtered water for about 10 minutes. Then, I mix it with other ingredients as described in step 2.

Agar-agar is packed with nutrients and vitamins such as:
- Vitamin E
- Vitamin K
- Zinc

- Copper
- Calcium
- Iron
- Magnesium
- Potassium
- Manganese.

It does not have a strong seaweed taste like for example, wakame, and is an excellent raw foods desserts and smoothie ingredients.

RECIPE#51 Raw Salad with Algae

Finally, talking about algae and seaweed let me introduce you to my raw salad with algae recipe!

Serves:2
Ingredients
- Half cup of dry agar-agar mixed with some tiny slices of alga wakame
- 1 red pepper
- 1 avocado
- Half onion
- ¼ cup of any nuts or seeds of your choice
- 2 big tomatoes
- 2 tablespoons of olive oil
- Himalaya salt
- OPTIONAL: a few slices of smoked salmon
- ¼ of iceberg lettuce
- Balsamic vinegar.

Instructions
1. Soak the algae in cold, filtered water for about 10 minutes.
2. Wash the iceberg lettuce and place on a kitchen cloth to dry the excess water.
3. In the meantime, wash and peel the pepper, avocado, tomato, and onion.
4. Slice the way you want to see them on your plate and mix with algae and iceberg lettuce (sliced).
5. Sprinkle over some olive oil, add some nuts, salt, and balsamic vinegar.

RECIPE#52 Spicy Eggplant Cream

This recipe can be served as a main dish or as a dip. I have also tried it as salad dressing. See which option suits you.

Serves-2

Ingredients

- 2 eggplants, peeled
- Filtered water
- 1 cup of almond milk or coconut milk
- Pinch of curry powder
- Pinch of chili powder
- Radish

Instructions

1. Chop the eggplants into small pieces and soak them in warm water (up to 30 degrees) until the water cools down.

2. In a blender, mix soaked eggplant chunks with some water (take about 1 cup of the water you were soaking them in) and coconut milk.

3. Blend until smoothed. Add some spices and Himalaya salt to taste.

4. Serve chilled with some sliced radishes.

Enjoy!

Additional Tips: How to Combine Raw Food Recipes from This Book with Other Diets As Well As Foods That Are Not Raw

1. If you are Paleo:
   - Use all those amazing salads, dips, and salsas to serve with your meat and fish. Focus on the recipes that are alkalizing to maintain a healthy balance. Too much meat in your diet is acid forming, this is why I strongly recommend you add as many raw foods as possible. This approach goes hand in hand with the real Paleolithic philosophy of eating only natural, unprocessed foods.
   - You can also serve your meat and fish in salads and soups—it can be an excellent combination!

2. If you are vegan:
   - Use grains such as quinoa, brown rice, millet, and amaranth and combine them with my recipes. Integral grains are an excellent combination with salads and soups.
   - Do the same with legumes such as lentils, chickpeas, beans, and adzuki.

3. If you are vegetarian:
   - The same as for vegans.
   - You can also experiment with a variety of natural kefirs, yoghurts and goat milk (even though it's animal milk, it's mildly alkalizing and much better for you than cow's milk).

- You can occasionally use boiled eggs in your raw salads and soups.
- You can occasionally use some organic goat's cheese in your raw foods salads and soups; it gives it a nice and creamy consistency.

4. If you are an alkaline diet lover:
   - Focus on raw foods that are alkalizing (about 70% of your diet) and the remaining 30% of fruits and vegetables can be acidic.
   - Make sure you keep hydrated, take advantage of raw foods juices and smoothies, and use fresh herbs with your recipes.
   - Eliminate caffeine, and try to switch to caffeine-free herbal teas such as kukicha and roibosh.

Conclusion

I hope that you enjoyed reading my recipes and have already chosen a few of them to try sometime soon. People who make at least 60-70% of their diet raw benefit from:

- Weight loss
- Brighter skin and healthier hair
- More energy levels
- More zest for life
- Less infections and colds
- Focused mind
  Use it as your MOTIVATION!

If you decide to do raw foods part-time (by saying part-time, I mean that you will be eating 50-70% raw), remember to make the remaining non-raw, or "cooked" part as healthy as possible, and eliminate all the processed foods. I think that as soon as you try eating raw at least part-time, and you go for natural, organic foods, you will start experiencing some really amazing health benefits that will make you hooked on a healthy lifestyle.

If you are new to raw foods, I suggest you invest some money in the following utensils and equipment; they will make your life easier and save your time:

- High speed blender
- Hand Blender (excellent when you travel)
- Juicer
- Spiral Slicer
- Food Processor
- Sprouter

To stay in touch with me, and be notified about more books & recipes to help you thrive, be sure to sign up for my alkaline wellness email newsletter (it's free).

www.HolisticWellnessProject.com/alkaline

If you have any problems, with your sign up, please e-mail me at:

Info@holisticwellnessproject.com

· ·

Finally, if you enjoyed my book and you feel like it has helped you and inspired you towards a healthier nutrition, please let others know! Simply post your review on Amazon.

Thanks in advance for your time and interest in my work.

It was a pleasure to "talk" to you,

I hope we "meet" again soon!

I wish you wellness, health, and success in whatever it is that you want to accomplish.

Marta

More Books in the Alkaline Lifestyle series

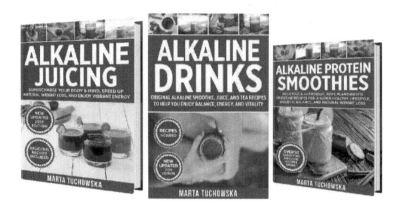

Now available on Amazon!

Manufactured by Amazon.ca
Bolton, ON

25900587R00068